CONSTIPATION TREATMENT HANDBOOK FOR BEGINNERS

An Exclusive Handbook Covering The Comprehension, Symptoms, Diagnosis, And Treatment Of Constipation, Including Both Medical And Alternative Remedies.

Vanessa Meza

Table of Contents

INTRODUCTION TO CONSTIPATION TREATMENT

A. Definition And Prevalence Of Constipation

B. Importance Of Addressing Constipation For Overall Health

C. Purpose Of The Book: Providing Effective Strategies And Remedies For Treating Constipation

A. Definition and Prevalence of Constipation:

Begin by defining constipation as a condition characterized by infrequent bowel movements or difficulty passing stool.

Provide statistics or prevalence rates to highlight the commonality of constipation, such as how many people are affected by it worldwide or in a specific demographic.

Explain common symptoms of constipation, such as straining during bowel movements, hard or lumpy stools, a feeling of incomplete evacuation, or abdominal discomfort.

B. Importance of Addressing Constipation for Overall Health:

Emphasize the significance of addressing constipation for overall health and well-being.

Discuss how untreated constipation can lead to complications such as hemorrhoids, anal fissures, fecal impaction, or even colorectal conditions.

Highlight the impact of constipation on quality of life, including discomfort, decreased appetite, and potential social embarrassment.

Mention the importance of maintaining regular bowel movements for proper digestion, nutrient absorption, and toxin removal.

C. Purpose of the Book: Providing Effective Strategies and Remedies for Treating Constipation:

Introduce the purpose of the book, which is to offer readers practical and effective strategies for managing and alleviating constipation.

Outline the scope of the book, including information on dietary changes, lifestyle modifications, natural remedies, and medical interventions.

Emphasize the book's goal of empowering readers with the knowledge and tools they need to address constipation effectively and improve their overall digestive health.

Highlight the importance of consulting with healthcare professionals for personalized advice and treatment recommendations.

CHAPTER ONE

UNDERSTANDING CONSTIPATION

A. Causes Of Constipation

1. **Dietary Factors**

2. **Lack Of Physical Activity**

3. **Medications And Medical Conditions**

B. Symptoms And Complications Of Chronic Constipation

A. Causes of Constipation:

Dietary Factors:

a. Discuss how a diet low in fiber can contribute to constipation, as fiber adds bulk to stool and promotes regular bowel movements.

b. Highlight specific foods that may exacerbate constipation, such as processed foods, dairy products, and refined carbohydrates.

c. Explain the importance of staying hydrated and consuming enough fluids to help soften stool and facilitate bowel movements.

Lack of Physical Activity:

a. Explain how a sedentary lifestyle can contribute to constipation by slowing down digestion and bowel motility. b. Emphasize the importance of regular exercise in promoting gastrointestinal health and maintaining healthy bowel habits.

Medications and Medical Conditions:
a. List common medications known to cause constipation as a side effect, such as certain pain relievers, antidepressants, and iron supplements.

b. Discuss how medical conditions like irritable bowel syndrome (IBS), hypothyroidism, diabetes, and neurological disorders can contribute to chronic constipation by affecting bowel function.

c. Mention the role of hormonal changes, such as those during pregnancy or menopause, in predisposing individuals to constipation.

B. Symptoms and Complications of Chronic Constipation:

Symptoms:

a. Describe the typical symptoms of chronic constipation, including infrequent bowel movements (fewer than three per week), straining during bowel movements, hard or lumpy stools, a sensation of incomplete evacuation, and abdominal discomfort or bloating.

b. Mention other symptoms that may accompany constipation, such as rectal bleeding, anal fissures, or hemorrhoids.

Complications:

a. Discuss potential complications that can arise from untreated or poorly managed chronic constipation, such as fecal impaction (a mass of hardened stool that cannot be expelled), which may require medical intervention for removal.

b. Highlight the risk of developing conditions like hemorrhoids, anal fissures, rectal prolapse, or diverticulosis due to chronic straining during bowel movements.

c. Emphasize the impact of chronic constipation on overall quality of life, including discomfort, decreased appetite, and psychological distress.

CHAPTER TWO

LIFESTYLE CHANGES FOR PREVENTING CONSTIPATION

A. Dietary Modifications

1. Increasing Fiber Intake

2. Staying Hydrated

3. Avoiding Certain Foods That Can Worsen Constipation

A. Dietary Modifications:

Increasing Fiber Intake: a. Encourage consuming a variety of high-fiber foods such as fruits, vegetables, whole grains, legumes, and nuts.

b. Emphasize the importance of gradually increasing fiber intake to prevent gastrointestinal discomfort or bloating.

c. Recommend specific fiber-rich foods like berries, prunes, apples, pears, broccoli, spinach, whole wheat bread, oats, and beans.

Staying Hydrated:

a. Stress the importance of adequate hydration for maintaining regular bowel movements and softening stool.

b. Advise drinking plenty of water throughout the day, aiming for at least 8-10 glasses or more depending on individual needs.

c. Suggest incorporating hydrating beverages like herbal teas, clear soups, and coconut water, while limiting intake of dehydrating beverages like alcohol and caffeinated drinks.

Avoiding Certain Foods that Can Worsen Constipation:

a. Identify foods that may exacerbate constipation, such as processed foods high in refined carbohydrates, fatty foods, and dairy products for individuals who are lactose intolerant.

b. Recommend reducing or avoiding intake of foods low in fiber and high in fat or sugar, which can slow down digestion and contribute to constipation.

c. Encourage mindful eating habits, including chewing food thoroughly and avoiding large meals that may overwhelm the digestive system.

B. EXERCISE AND PHYSICAL ACTIVITY

1. Importance Of Regular Exercise In Promoting Bowel Movements

2. Recommended Types Of Exercises For Relieving Constipation

Importance of Regular Exercise in Promoting Bowel Movements: a. Explain how regular exercise helps stimulate bowel movements by increasing intestinal muscle contractions and promoting the movement of waste through the digestive tract.

b. Emphasize the role of physical activity in improving overall gastrointestinal motility and reducing the risk of constipation.

c. Highlight the benefits of exercise for maintaining a healthy weight, managing stress, and enhancing overall well-being, all of which can indirectly contribute to better bowel function.

Recommended Types of Exercises for Relieving Constipation:

a. Aerobic Exercise:

Recommend aerobic exercises such as brisk walking, jogging, cycling, swimming, or dancing, which help increase heart rate and stimulate intestinal activity.

Encourage engaging in aerobic activities for at least 30 minutes most days of the week to promote regular bowel movements.

b. Core-Strengthening Exercises:

Suggest incorporating core-strengthening exercises like planks, bridges, yoga, or Pilates, which help improve abdominal muscle tone and support healthy bowel function.

Emphasize the importance of maintaining proper form and technique to avoid exacerbating any existing gastrointestinal issues.

 c. Stretching and Yoga:

Advocate for stretching exercises and yoga poses that target the abdominal area and promote relaxation, such as forward bends, twists, and gentle twists.

Highlight the stress-reducing benefits of yoga and its potential to alleviate tension in the digestive system, which can help relieve constipation.

d. Pelvic Floor Exercises:

Recommend pelvic floor exercises, also known as Kegel exercises, to strengthen the muscles that control bowel movements and prevent fecal incontinence.

Explain how regular practice of pelvic floor exercises can improve bowel control and alleviate symptoms of constipation, especially in individuals with weakened pelvic floor muscles.

C. ESTABLISHING HEALTHY BOWEL HABITS

1. Regular Bowel Movements Schedule

2. Proper Toilet Posture And Techniques

Regular Bowel Movements Schedule:

a. Stress the importance of establishing a consistent daily routine for bowel movements, ideally at the same time each day.

b. Encourage individuals to listen to their body's natural cues and respond promptly when the urge to have a bowel movement arises.

c. Recommend allocating sufficient time for bowel movements without feeling rushed or interrupted, as this can help promote complete evacuation and reduce the risk of constipation.

d. Advise against ignoring the urge to defecate or delaying bowel movements, as this can lead to stool retention and exacerbate constipation.

Proper Toilet Posture and Techniques:
a. Explain the significance of proper toilet posture in facilitating easier

bowel movements and reducing strain on the pelvic floor muscles. b. Recommend using a squatting position on the toilet, either by elevating the feet with a footstool or using a specialized squatting platform, to mimic the natural squatting posture adopted by our ancestors. c. Emphasize the importance of maintaining good posture while seated on the toilet, with the knees higher than the hips and the spine straight, to promote optimal alignment and reduce abdominal pressure.

d. Encourage relaxation techniques such as deep breathing or visualization exercises to help ease tension in the pelvic floor muscles and encourage bowel movements. e. Advise against straining or bearing down excessively during bowel movements, as this can increase the risk of pelvic floor dysfunction and other complications.

CHAPTER TWO

NATURAL REMEDIES FOR CONSTIPATION RELIEF

A. HERBAL REMEDIES AND SUPPLEMENTS

1. **Psyllium Husk**

2. **Senna**

3. **Magnesium Supplements**

B. HOME REMEDIES

1. **Warm Water With Lemon**

2. **Prune Juice**

3. **Castor Oil**

C. PROBIOTICS AND THEIR ROLE IN MAINTAINING GUT HEALTH

A. Herbal Remedies and Supplements:

Psyllium Husk:

a. Explain how psyllium husk, a soluble fiber derived from the Plantago ovata plant, can help relieve constipation by adding bulk to stool and promoting regular bowel movements.

 b. Recommend taking psyllium husk supplements with plenty of water to prevent potential choking or gastrointestinal obstruction.

c. Advise starting with a low dose and gradually increasing as needed, while monitoring for any adverse effects such as bloating or gas.

Senna: a. Discuss how senna, a natural laxative derived from the leaves and pods of the Senna alexandrina plant, works by stimulating bowel contractions and promoting evacuation.

b. Caution against long-term or excessive use of senna, as it may lead to dependence or electrolyte imbalances.

c. Recommend using senna-based products sparingly and under the guidance of a healthcare professional, especially for individuals with certain medical conditions or taking other medications.

Magnesium Supplements:

a. Explain how magnesium supplements can help relieve constipation by drawing water into the intestines and promoting bowel motility.

b. Recommend magnesium citrate or magnesium oxide supplements as preferred forms for constipation relief.

c. Advise against exceeding recommended dosages of magnesium supplements, as excessive intake may cause diarrhea or other gastrointestinal symptoms.

B. Home Remedies:

Warm Water with Lemon:

a. Suggest starting the day with a glass of warm water mixed with freshly squeezed lemon juice to help stimulate digestion and bowel movements. b. Explain how lemon juice's acidic properties may help cleanse the digestive system and promote bowel regularity.

Prune Juice: a. Highlight the natural laxative effects of prune juice, which is high in fiber, sorbitol, and natural sugars.

b. Recommend drinking prune juice in moderation, as excessive consumption may lead to diarrhea or abdominal discomfort.

Castor Oil:

a. Discuss the traditional use of castor oil as a natural laxative, which works by stimulating smooth muscle contractions in the intestines. b. Caution against using castor oil as a first-line treatment for constipation, as it may cause cramping, nausea, and diarrhea.

C. Probiotics and Their Role in Maintaining Gut Health:

a. Explain how probiotics, beneficial bacteria found in certain foods and supplements, can help maintain a healthy balance of gut microbiota and promote regular bowel movements.

b. Recommend consuming probiotic-rich foods such as yogurt, kefir, sauerkraut, and kimchi, or taking probiotic supplements with strains known to support digestive health.

c. Discuss the importance of selecting high-quality probiotic products with evidence-based strains and appropriate potency levels.

CHAPTER THREE

MEDICAL TREATMENTS FOR SEVERE CONSTIPATION

A. Over-The-Counter Laxatives

B. Prescription Medications For Chronic Constipation

C. Procedures And Surgeries For Severe Cases

A. Over-the-Counter Laxatives: Bulk-forming Laxatives:

a. Explain how bulk-forming laxatives, such as psyllium husk or methylcellulose, work by absorbing water in the intestines, softening stool, and increasing bulk to promote bowel movements.

b. Recommend bulk-forming laxatives as a first-line treatment for mild to moderate constipation, emphasizing the importance of adequate fluid intake to prevent intestinal obstruction.

Osmotic Laxatives:

a. Discuss how osmotic laxatives, such as polyethylene glycol (PEG) or magnesium hydroxide, work by drawing water into the intestines, softening stool, and promoting bowel movements.

b. Advise using osmotic laxatives for short-term relief of constipation, cautioning against prolonged use due to the risk of electrolyte imbalances or dehydration.

Stimulant Laxatives: a. Explain how stimulant laxatives, such as bisacodyl or senna, work by stimulating intestinal contractions and increasing bowel motility. b. Recommend using stimulant laxatives sparingly and under the guidance of a healthcare professional, as long-term use may lead to dependence or bowel dysfunction.

B. Prescription Medications for Chronic Constipation:

Prokinetic Agents:

a. Discuss how prokinetic agents, such as prucalopride or tegaserod, work by enhancing intestinal motility and accelerating transit time to relieve chronic constipation.

b. Highlight the importance of careful dosing and monitoring for potential side effects, especially in individuals with underlying gastrointestinal conditions.

Lubricant Laxatives:

a. Explain how lubricant laxatives, such as mineral oil, work by coating the stool and intestinal walls, facilitating passage and reducing straining.

 b. Caution against using mineral oil as a long-term solution due to the risk of aspiration pneumonia and interference with nutrient absorption.

Prescription-strength Osmotic Laxatives:

 a. Discuss how prescription-strength osmotic laxatives, such as lactulose or prescription-grade PEG, may be recommended for individuals with severe or refractory constipation. b. Emphasize the importance of proper dosing and monitoring for electrolyte imbalances or other adverse effects, especially in vulnerable populations.

C. Procedures and Surgeries for Severe Cases:

Manual Disimpaction: a. Describe manual disimpaction as a procedure performed by a healthcare professional to manually remove impacted stool from the rectum and lower colon. b. Explain that manual disimpaction may be necessary in cases of severe fecal impaction that do not respond to other treatments.

Surgical Interventions: a. Discuss surgical options such as colectomy (partial or total removal of the colon) or rectopexy (surgical fixation of the rectum) for individuals with severe refractory constipation or underlying structural abnormalities. b. Emphasize that surgical interventions are typically considered as a last resort when all other treatments have failed, and they carry risks and potential complications that must be weighed carefully.

CHAPTER FOUR

MANAGING CONSTIPATION IN SPECIAL POPULATIONS

A. Constipation In Children

1. Causes And Treatment Strategies Tailored For Children

B. Constipation During Pregnancy

1. Safe Remedies And Lifestyle Changes For Pregnant Women

C. Constipation In The Elderly

1. Unique Challenges And Considerations For Managing Constipation In Older Adults

A. Constipation in Children:

Causes and Treatment Strategies Tailored for Children:

a. Discuss common causes of constipation in children, such as diet low in fiber, inadequate fluid intake, withholding stools due to fear or pain, or medical conditions like Hirschsprung's disease or cystic fibrosis.

b. Recommend age-appropriate dietary modifications, such as increasing fiber-rich foods like fruits, vegetables, and whole grains, and ensuring adequate hydration with water or diluted fruit juices.

c. Encourage regular physical activity and toilet training techniques that promote relaxation and comfortable bowel movements.

d. Discuss the importance of establishing a regular toilet routine and providing positive reinforcement for successful bowel movements.

e. Highlight the use of pediatric-friendly laxatives or stool softeners under the guidance of a pediatrician, avoiding stimulant laxatives unless recommended by a healthcare professional.

B. Constipation During Pregnancy:

Safe Remedies and Lifestyle Changes for Pregnant Women:

a.	Acknowledge the common occurrence of constipation during pregnancy, attributed to hormonal changes, increased pressure on the intestines from the growing uterus, and prenatal vitamins containing iron.

b. Recommend dietary modifications similar to those for the general population, emphasizing high-fiber foods, adequate hydration, and regular physical activity, while considering individual dietary preferences and tolerances.

c.   Suggest   safe   over-the-counter laxatives such as bulk-forming agents or osmotic laxatives under the guidance of a healthcare provider, avoiding stimulant laxatives or herbal remedies that may pose risks during pregnancy.

d. Encourage prenatal care providers to monitor and address constipation as part of routine prenatal care, providing reassurance and support for pregnant women experiencing discomfort or concerns.

C. Constipation in the Elderly:

Unique Challenges and Considerations for Managing Constipation in Older Adults:

a. Recognize the prevalence of constipation in the elderly population, attributed to factors such as decreased mobility, medications with constipating side effects, dietary changes, and age-related changes in gastrointestinal function.

b. Emphasize the importance of addressing underlying medical conditions or medications contributing to constipation through comprehensive geriatric assessment and medication review.

 c. Recommend lifestyle modifications tailored to the individual's abilities and preferences, such as gentle exercise or physical activity, hydration, and dietary adjustments with consideration of chewing difficulties or dental problems.

d. Discuss the use of laxatives or stool softeners cautiously in older adults, considering potential risks of dehydration, electrolyte imbalance, or impaired bowel function, and advocating for regular monitoring and adjustment of medications as needed.

PSYCHOLOGICAL ASPECTS OF CONSTIPATION

A. Stress And Its Impact On Bowel Movements

B. Behavioral Therapies For Managing Stress-Related Constipation

C. Mindfulness And Relaxation Techniques For Improving Bowel Function

A. Stress and Its Impact on Bowel Movements:

Explain the bidirectional relationship between stress and bowel movements, highlighting how stress can affect the functioning of the digestive system.

Discuss the physiological mechanisms by which stress can influence bowel habits, such as activating the body's fight-or-flight response, which can slow down digestion and intestinal motility.

Emphasize the role of the gut-brain axis in connecting the central nervous system with the enteric nervous system, which controls gastrointestinal functions, and how stress can disrupt this communication, leading to symptoms like constipation.

B. Behavioral Therapies for Managing Stress-Related Constipation:

Cognitive Behavioral Therapy (CBT):

a. Introduce CBT as a therapeutic approach aimed at identifying and changing negative thought patterns and behaviors that contribute to stress and constipation.

b. Discuss how CBT techniques, such as cognitive restructuring, relaxation training, and stress management strategies, can help individuals cope with stress and improve bowel function.

Biofeedback Therapy:

a. Explain how biofeedback therapy involves using electronic sensors to monitor physiological functions, such as muscle activity in the pelvic floor, and providing visual or auditory feedback to help individuals learn to control these functions.

b. Highlight the potential effectiveness of biofeedback therapy in treating pelvic floor dysfunction and functional constipation by teaching individuals how to relax pelvic muscles and coordinate bowel movements.

C. Mindfulness and Relaxation Techniques for Improving Bowel Function:

Mindfulness Meditation:

a. Describe mindfulness meditation as a practice that involves paying nonjudgmental attention to the present moment, including bodily sensations, thoughts, and emotions.

b. Discuss how mindfulness-based interventions, such as mindfulness-based stress reduction (MBSR) or mindfulness-based cognitive therapy (MBCT), can help individuals reduce stress, increase body awareness, and improve self-regulation of bowel function.

Progressive Muscle Relaxation (PMR):
a. Introduce PMR as a relaxation technique that involves systematically tensing and relaxing different muscle groups in the body to promote physical and mental relaxation.

b. Explain how PMR can help individuals reduce muscle tension, alleviate stress, and promote smoother bowel movements by enhancing overall relaxation and reducing stress-related symptoms.

CONCLUSION

A. Recap Of Key Points Discussed In The Book

B. Encouragement For Readers To Take Proactive Steps In Addressing Constipation

C. Hope For A Healthier And Happier Life Free From The Discomfort Of Constipation

A. Recap of Key Points Discussed in the Book:

Understanding Constipation: We explored the definition, prevalence, and causes of constipation, highlighting the importance of addressing this common digestive issue.

Lifestyle Changes: We discussed dietary modifications, exercise, establishing healthy bowel habits, and natural remedies for preventing and managing constipation.

Medical Treatments: We covered over-the-counter and prescription medications, as well as procedures and surgeries for severe cases of constipation.

Managing Constipation in Special Populations: We provided tailored strategies for children, pregnant women, and the elderly, recognizing their unique challenges and considerations.

B. Encouragement for Readers to Take Proactive Steps in Addressing Constipation:

I encourage readers to take proactive steps in managing their bowel health. By incorporating the strategies outlined in this book, including dietary changes, exercise, stress management techniques, and appropriate medical interventions, individuals can effectively prevent and alleviate constipation, leading to improved overall well-being.

C. Hope for a Healthier and Happier Life Free from the Discomfort of Constipation:

Lastly, I offer hope for a healthier and happier life free from the discomfort of constipation. By prioritizing bowel health and adopting healthy habits, individuals can experience greater comfort, energy, and vitality. Remember, you have the power to take control of your digestive health and enjoy a life without the limitations of constipation.

www.ingramcontent.com/pod-product-compliance
Lightning Source LLC
Chambersburg PA
CBHW071216260726
48653CB00041B/880